One Touch Healing

Mildred Carter • Tammy Weber

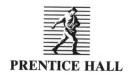

PRENTICE HALL

Printed in the United States of America

10 9 8 7 6 5 4 3 2

This book is a reference work based on research by the author. Any techniques and suggestions are to be used at the reader's sole discretion. The opinions expressed herein are not necessarily those of or endorsed by the publisher. The directions stated in this book are in no way to be considered as a substitute for consultation with a duly licensed doctor.

Photography by Jennifer Rodgers

ISBN 0-13-974197-6

ATTENTION: CORPORATIONS AND SCHOOLS

Prentice Hall books are available at quantity discounts with bulk purchase for educational, business, or sales promotional use. For information, please write to: Prentice Hall Special Sales, 240 Frisch Court, Paramus, New Jersey 07652. Please supply: title of book, ISBN, quantity, how the book will be used, date needed.

PRENTICE HALL
Paramus, NJ 07652

A Simon & Schuster Company

On the World Wide Web at http://www.phdirect.com

Prentice Hall International (UK) Limited, *London*
Prentice Hall of Australia Pty. Limited, *Sydney*
Prentice Hall Canada Inc., *Toronto*
Prentice Hall Hispanoamericana, S.A., *Mexico*
Prentice Hall of India Private Limited, *New Delhi*
Prentice Hall of Japan, Inc., *Tokyo*
Simon & Schuster Asia Pte. Ltd., *Singapore*
Editora Prentice Hall do Brasil, Ltda., *Rio de Janeiro*

Contents

How Reflexology Works to Help the Body Heal Itself

More than twenty million Americans have seen the effectiveness of reflexology on TV and have read of this natural technique of healing in many national magazines as well as in most newspapers. It is sometimes described under different names, but all these methods use the technique of pressing on certain points of the body.

I have proved beyond any doubt whatever the healing power of reflex massage in my books *Hand Reflexology: Key to Perfect Health* and *Helping Yourself with Foot Reflexology.*

Now we will take you a step further with the wonders of body massage which will also bring miracles of healing into your life and the lives of those you love.

Body reflexology will start the functioning of many processes throughout the whole body and leave nothing unattended when you follow the directions given.

You will release the healing power of the lymphatic system by opening up the flow of lymph fluid into damaged areas. You will speed up the healing forces by activating the nervous system when you massage the reflexes as directed and balance the vital energies among all the various systems.

Glance for a moment at Diagram 1. Notice how energy and circulation are slowed down when there is blockage in the line. We start health flowing back into our bodies by breaking up this blockage and letting the life energy flow freely to all parts of the body.

1

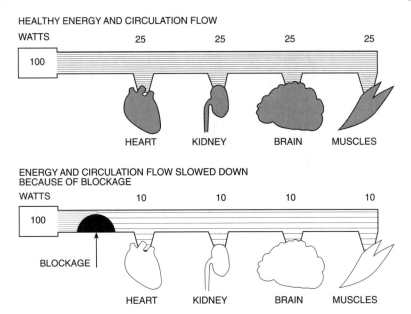

HEALTHY ENERGY AND CIRCULATION FLOW
WATTS   25   25   25   25
100

HEART   KIDNEY   BRAIN   MUSCLES

ENERGY AND CIRCULATION FLOW SLOWED DOWN
BECAUSE OF BLOCKAGE
WATTS   10   10   10   10
100

BLOCKAGE

HEART   KIDNEY   BRAIN   MUSCLES

Diagram 1

A tender spot any place on your body indicates a point of congestion in the energy lines, which in turn means trouble in some area that may be far removed from the tender point.

Now you can see why reflexology works such miracles of healing. This simple miracle of magic healing has been overlooked for many years because of its very simplicity.

HOW REFLEXOLOGY WORKS

The press of a finger on a certain "button" (nerve ending) on the body may result in an odd tingling sensation in quite a different area, and you will know that the reflex button is connected with this remote part. Hold it for a few seconds; if it is sensitive, press it several times. You now have proof that the healing pressure on a reflex is getting through to the source of the trouble.

Sometimes the tingling will be felt where you least expect it. This doesn't always happen, but when it does you will be aware that you have discovered a life-giving current of health. It is this reward that makes reflex massage so valuable. It covers all parts of the body and brings them under control. It keeps corrosion from forming and causing trouble later on.

Don't be impatient. You must keep in mind that it has taken a long time for you to get into your present condition. Now you must give nature some time to correct it, although often the improvement is so rapid that it does seem like a miracle.

In some cases it is necessary to use prolonged stimulation to alleviate the pain, sometimes from twenty minutes to an hour. So don't give up if the pain does not subside immediately. It will work!

TREAT THE SLIGHTEST TWINGE OF PAIN

Whenever you feel a pain anywhere in your body, even the slightest twinge of a pain, no matter where it is located, press and massage it *immediately*! It is the body's method of sending you a signal via the reflexes that there is trouble. Someplace there is a blockage causing malfunctioning to a certain area in the body. It may be far removed from the messenger sending the signal, but press the button now and you may prevent future illness from striking unexpectedly later on. Listen to your body. You will always get a warning signal before illness strikes, so heed it as you would a red light at a street crossing. *Stop* and press the reflex button, and you will continue to live free from illness.

Techniques for Pressing Reflexes All Over the Body

In describing how to use reflexes found all over the body, it is best to start with those found in the hands and feet.

Place your thumb in the center of your palm or in the center of the bottom of your foot and, with a rotating motion, press and roll the thumb as if you were trying to break up lumpy sugar. Do this about five times; then move to another spot. You can tell which reflex you are massaging by studying Diagrams 2, 3, 4, and 5. You are *not* to rub the *skin* but the reflexes *under the skin*. Use this method for massaging reflexes, except where instructed to hold a steady pressure.

A more advanced method of massaging the hands and the feet involves starting to rub the thumb or the big toe, then completely massaging every finger and every toe, searching for tender reflexes. Don't just use your fingers here. Use a device like a pencil or little hand reflex probe. Roll this between every toe on both sides and also between every finger. You will be amazed at the "ouch" spots you will discover in these areas.

In Diagrams 6A, 6D, and 6E, you will find that there are also important reflexes on the tops of the feet and on the backs of the hands. Be sure to massage these reflex buttons to stimulate many areas in the body. Hold a steady, firm pressure for a slow count of seven, and then release for a count of three. Do this three times more on the calves of the legs for about 15 minutes to alleviate pain throughout the entire body. See Diagram 6H.

4

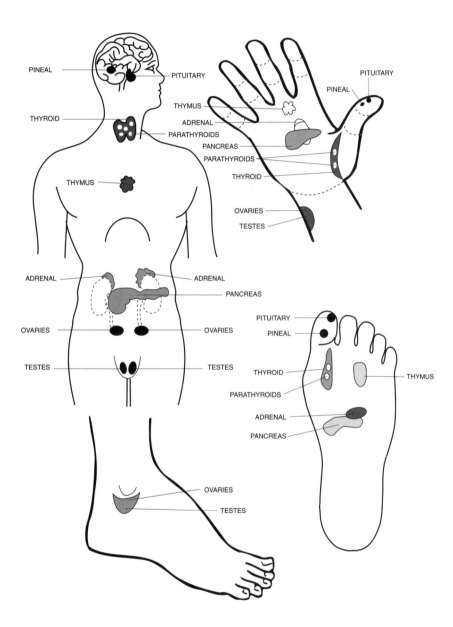

Diagram 2

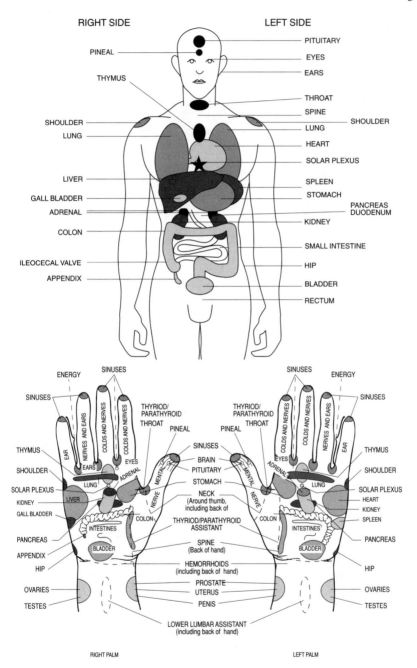

Diagram 3

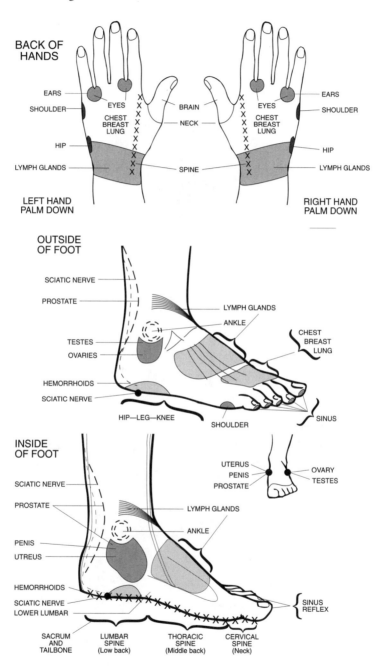

Diagram 4

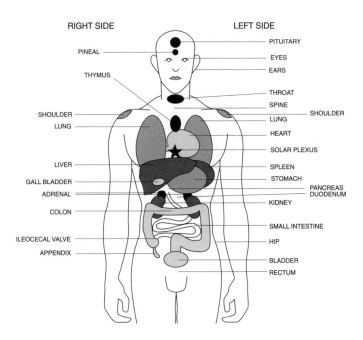

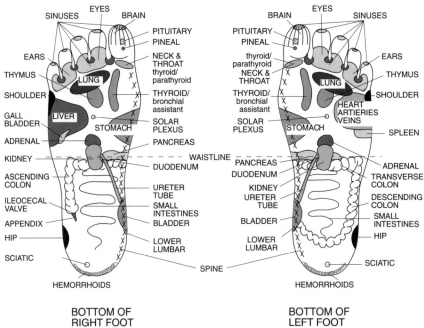

Diagram 5

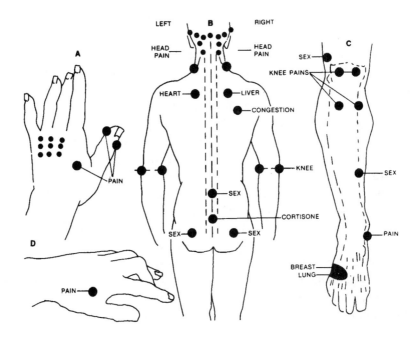

This diagram shows several pain control reflex buttons that are stimulated by pressure that causes them to release natural pain-inhibiting chemicals in the brain called "endorphines." Also shown are energy-stimulating reflex buttons in various locations.

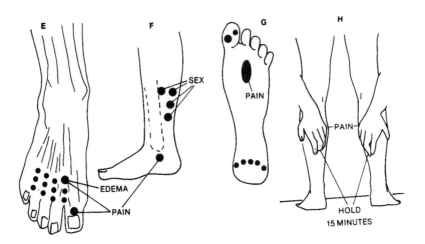

Diagram 6

BODY REFLEXES

You can see by studying the diagrams that follow that, unlike the reflexes in the hands and the feet, body reflexes do not always follow a straight meridian line. There are *several* reflex points located in certain areas of the body that will stimulate renewed life to more than one malfunctioning area.

So, we will have to use a somewhat new technique when using the body reflexes. Because these reflex buttons are sometimes in hard-to-massage areas, it is difficult to give simple directions.

By studying the diagrams, you will see what I mean. In Diagram 12, notice how many reflexes are located in just a portion of the head. How are you going to find a specific button? Hence some new techniques come into play. You will find photos of most of them. Sometimes it may be necessary to ask another person for help.

Look at Diagrams 7 and 8. You will see reflex points scattered over various parts of the body. Now turn to Diagrams 9, 10, and 11. Many of you are not familiar with the glands and organs within the body; I would like you to study the positions of these glands and organs so you will be able to associate them with certain reflex buttons when you are instructed to massage them for specific ailments.

HOW TO WORK BODY REFLEXES FOR THE MOST EFFECTIVE RESULTS

Look at Diagrams 3 and 5. Note how the reflex buttons are located more or less over the glands and organs they represent. To press these specific reflex points, use the middle finger, which has the strongest energy flow, or use the four-finger method, which sometimes seems to have the power of a laser beam. There are several ways in which you can massage (or work) these sensitive reflex buttons. All reflex buttons not named on the charts are energy stimulants and important to many areas of the body. You will find many tender reflex buttons that are not marked. Don't let this worry you. If they are sending an "ouch" signal, this means that some place in your body is in trouble and is asking for your help. So work it out.

It is best to start by massaging the *important* reflexes located in various places over the entire body.

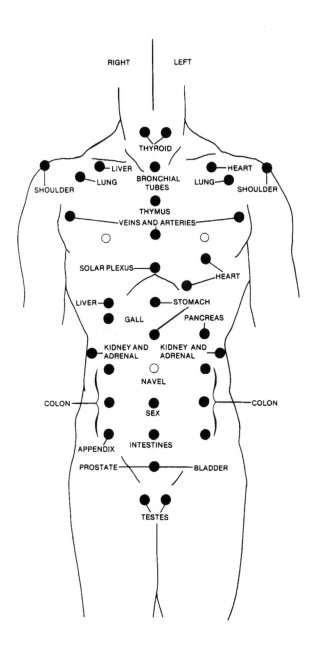

Diagram 7

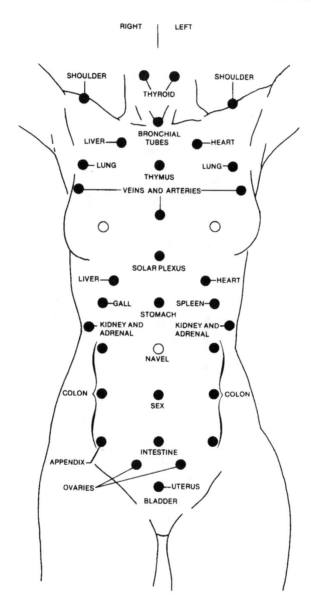

Diagram 8

MIRROR IMAGE

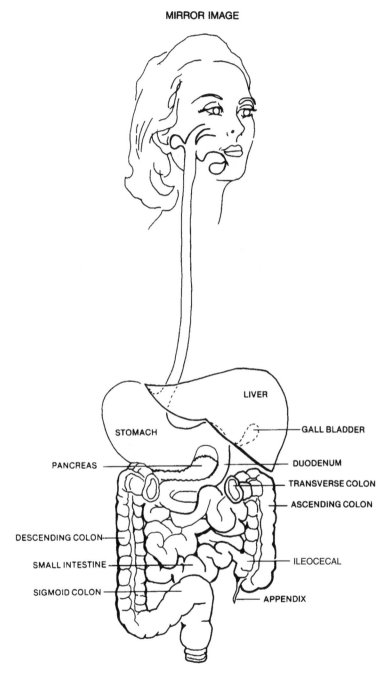

Diagram 9

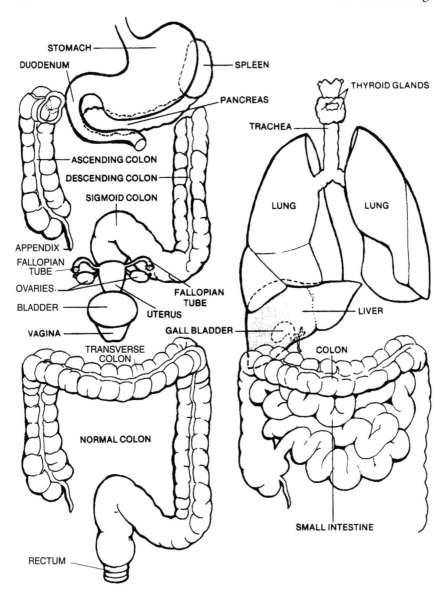

Diagram 10

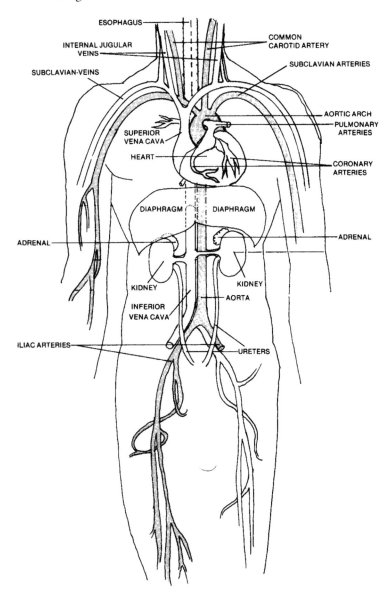

Diagram 11

Use the middle finger to press lightly on each reflex button. If it is painful, you will know that there is congestion somewhere. Let us say that you find a painful button over the stomach area. This does not necessarily mean that the stomach is the organ in trouble. When you look at Diagrams 7 and 8, you can see that tender reflexes could be sending out pain signals from other malfunctioning nerves or tissue in a congested area. If it hurts when pressed, assume that there is a blocked line that is slowing down the electrical life force to a congested area. Hold pressure on this reflex button until the hurt subsides or for seven seconds at a time. Keep in mind that you are doing more than diagnosing areas of malfunction when you massage these reflexes that are giving you warning signals of congestion or malfunctioning of a certain organ, gland, or tissue. You are also treating the *ailment*, restoring health by releasing the blockage to the energy field.

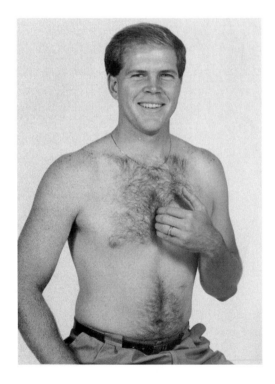

Photo 1: Position for pressing reflexes to the thymus, veins, and arteries.

How to Use Special Exercises to Stimulate the Reflexes on the Head

Several diagrams of the head are included in this section. As you study them, you will be amazed at the many reflexes you will find and how they are related to all parts of your body.

When I give you specific directions on how to stimulate the reflexes, you will better understand their importance. You need not learn where all these reflexes are located by sight, but with a little practice you will learn their approximate locations by feel. This will hold true in most cases throughout this book. Study the diagrams and photos as we progress.

TECHNIQUE FOR MASSAGING THE REFLEXES ON THE HEAD

Study Diagrams 12, 13, and 14. Take note of how many important reflexes are located here. You do not need to remember where they are located; I will point these out to you as we need them further on in the book. I just want you to familiarize yourself with the importance of the different techniques of working the reflexes in the head.

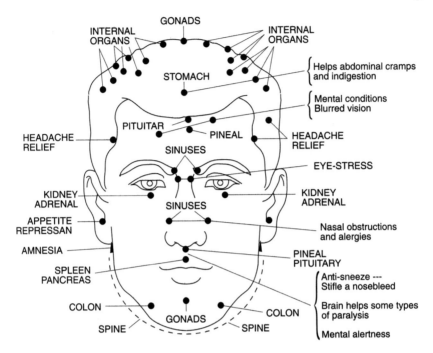

Diagram 12

Use your fingers to find special areas on the head. In Diagram 12, notice on the very center of the top of the head we find the reflexes to the reproductive organs. Down toward the forehead is the reflex to the stomach. Under the nose we find the reflex to the pineal and pituitary, then the spleen, and then the pancreas reflexes. Straight down from these reflexes we find the gonad reflexes on the chin. This seems to be on the center meridian line that runs through the body.

One way to massage these reflexes is to use the center finger, which is called the fire finger because it sends out energy more strongly than the other fingers. Press it on the center of the forehead just below the hair line. With a pressing, rolling motion feel for a sensitive spot. Do not rub the skin; rather, rub the bone area under the skin very gently. Now, move the finger down to the center of the forehead and feel for another tender button, which will be a reflex to the pineal (commonly known as the third eye). Halfway between this spot and the bridge of the nose is another sensitive reflex that needs massage. This reflex affects the sinuses.

Back of the Head

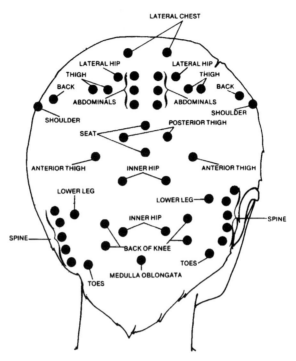

Diagram 13

Massaging Only Certain Reflexes

This is one way to massage specific reflex buttons on the head. But you do not need to massage each and every one of these reflexes unless told to do so for a specific purpose. Other and easier methods of stimulating all these head and face reflexes more fully will be described later. But, for now, do note that head massages are very important.

Look at Diagram 13, illustrating the back of the head. Notice all the reflexes located here. Now go to Diagram 14 to see the location of the reflexes on the side of the head. You may have to refer back to these charts now and then when following directions for treating mal-functioning areas elsewhere in the body. We will use the three different methods of stimulation shown in Photos 2, 3, and 4.

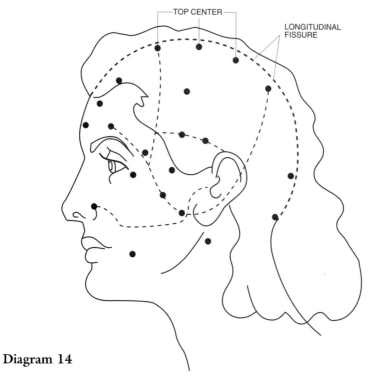

Diagram 14

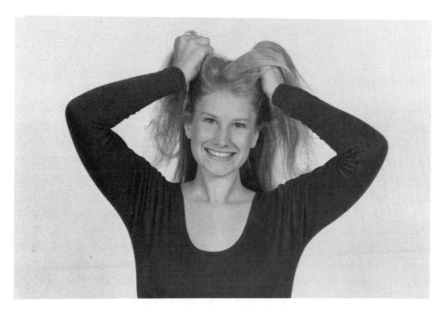

Photo 2: Pulling hair stimulates the whole body, helps indigestion, hangovers, etc.

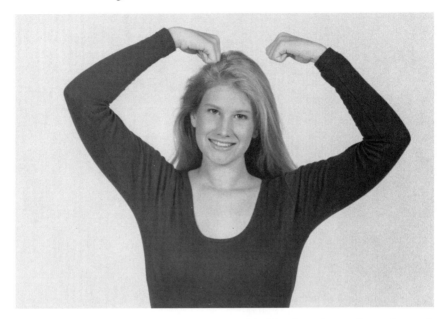

Photo 3: Lightly tap head to promote bladder function and good sexual activity, as well as other benefits.

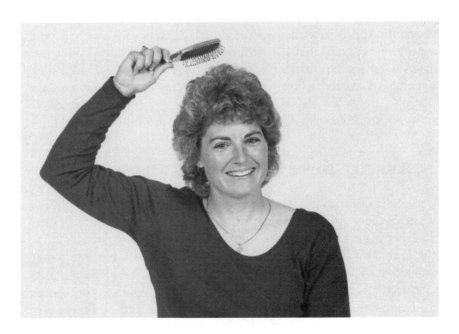

Photo 4: Tapping the head and body with the wire brush stimulates all the body reflexes.

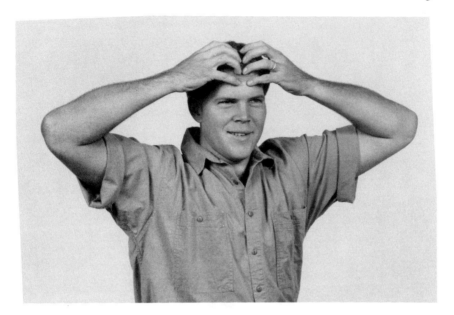

Photo 5: Position for working reflexes on head and forehead.

A car door once slammed on my head (my head had been caught between the top of the car and the door). I felt funny and had odd headaches for several days. I felt that the cranial bones had been jammed together. No doctors in the area were familiar with adjusting the skull, so I started to press and pull the cranial bones myself (see Photo 5). After a few days I felt better and the uncomfortable sensations in my head stopped. This was several years ago, and I still feel fine.

THE ALL-IMPORTANT MEDULLA OBLONGATA

The medulla oblongata is a reflex button that we will use throughout. It is one of the magic buttons that will start your power generator into action. It will enable you to open up the electrical channels to all parts of the body. It will bring you release from daily nervous tensions when you need it. This button will generate almost instant energy. You decide on the action you want, and in seconds it is yours to command. This magic reflex button can be used at any time and in almost any location without anyone knowing what you are doing.

In Diagram 13 notice the button located in the hollow at the base of the skull on the back of the head. This is the medulla oblongata, a vitality-generating reflex button. It is the enlarged portion of the spinal cord, just after it enters the cranium. It is a giant controlling agent containing the cardiovascular center and the respirator center. It controls blood pressure and the dilation and constriction of blood vessels. It controls postural balance and the reflexes concerned with swallowing, vomiting, and many other actions. Even though the spinal cord is located on the inside of the skull, you will cause reactions whenever you apply any type of reflex therapy to it. The entire body network funnels impulses into the spinal cord. These messages are relayed to the power-manufacturing centers of the brain and body. The messages are sent to all the endocrine glands.

The medulla oblongata reflex will give you instant go-power when it is needed. It is a very important reflex button and will be referred to many times, so it is important that you learn the best technique for massaging it.

Technique of Reflex Massage

To turn on this sensational dynamo of action, find a little hollow between two muscle attachments at the base of the skull. See medulla oblongata, Diagram 13. Use either the middle finger of one hand or the middle fingers of both hands. You will have to use the method that is easiest for you. Now, put the finger or fingers into the hollow area and press. Is it painful? Feel it! Press it! Massage it! This is the fantastic magic reflex button that can give you the unlimited energy and go-power that everyone needs in these busy, stress-filled days.

SPECIAL BODY WARMER REFLEXES

As you study Diagram 14, you will see special points marked in various places on the side of the head. These are known as neurovascular receptors. I call them the body warmer reflexes to keep them simple and easy to remember. Each of these special reflexes is in a relative position. Remember that all heads are not the same shape, so you have to learn the approximate areas by searching for tender or sensitive points. With practice, you will learn to find them on yourself and others quite easily by reaching and feeling with your fingers. See Photos 5, 6, 7, 8, and 9 for different positions used to massage these body warmer reflexes on the head. These body warmer reflexes keep the lines open to special heaters in various parts of the body.

Let us liken the body warmers to little electric heaters that control the temperature of the entire body. If you are unable to adjust to temperature changes in the weather, some of your body heaters are not functioning properly and need to be reactivated.

These body warmers gather and regulate the energy of the digestive, sexual, and respiratory organs, and others. They work in cooperation with the lungs, the small intestines, the kidneys, the heart, and the sex organs.

The meridian of the body warmers begins at the root of the nail of the little finger and ascends up the back part of the body. If you will look once more at Diagram 14, you will better understand how the exercises that I give you to massage the head will help stimulate most, if not all, of the body warmer reflexes in the whole body.

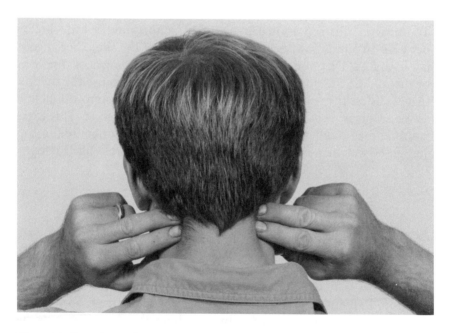

Photo 6: Pressing reflexes on the edge of the skull for headache and other complaints.

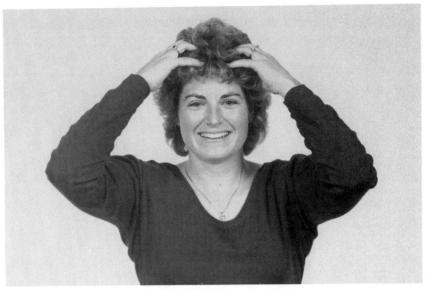

Photo 7: Position for pressing reflexes on top of head to energize areas in the whole body. Also benefits mental conditions.

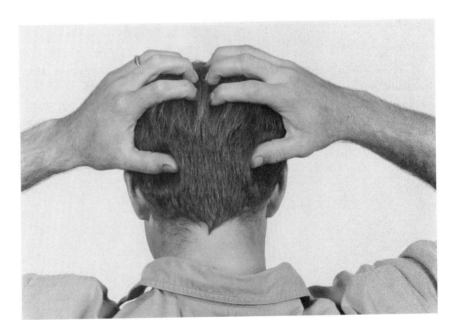

Photo 8: Position for massaging reflexes on back of head to energize many areas of the body.

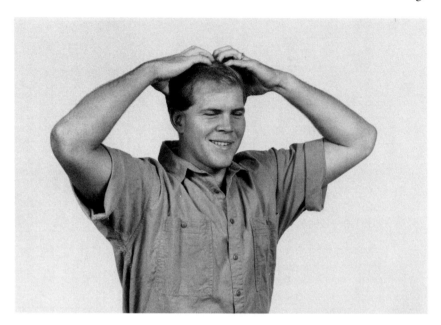

Photo 9: Shows position for stimulating the thyroid, gonads, lungs, and heart.

As we work the reflexes in other places of the body, we automatically press on and massage many of the body warmers without having to learn their exact locations. Keep in mind that if you find a tender reflex, no matter what part of the body it is getting a distress signal from, you should press and hold it until the hurt subsides.

How to Use Reflexology on the Ears

As you can see in Diagram 15, there are many important reflexes in the ears. They will stimulate a renewed flow of life force into every part of your body when pressed, pulled, and massaged. The ears, like the hands and the feet, have reflexes for the entire body. Because of the relationship of the reflexes in the ears to the rest of the body, reflex massage of the ears can help to correct many symptoms of malfunctioning organs.

THE EAR AND ITS ACUPOINTS

The ear is a complex sense organ endowed with a hundred acupoints. Its accessibility makes it ideal for the acupuncturist, who uses needles for stimulation to promote health in the rest of the body.

We have now learned to use the fingers to stimulate these sensitive reflexes. People twist, pull, and pinch their ears unconsciously, especially the earlobes, when something perplexing bothers them. Thus, instinctively, people reinvent this wonderful healing technique.

Because there are some one hundred reflexes in the ears, it is almost impossible to pinpoint all of them, so let us do a few exercises to stimulate as many of them as possible.

See Photo 10. Place the fingers behind the ears and flatten them forward against the side of the head. Holding the ear with the third, fourth, and fifth fingers, tap the index finger on the ear to get a drum sound. Do this about five times to stimulate the gallbladder.

THE EAR

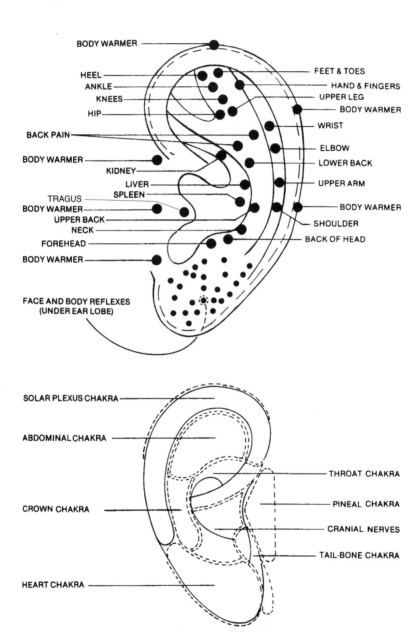

Diagram 15

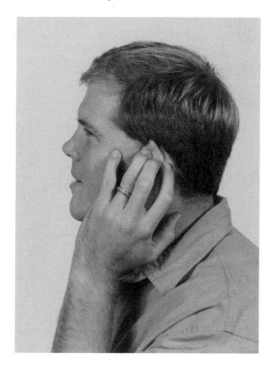

Photo 10: Bending the ear forward for tapping.

Now, place the cupped hand over one ear and tap gently with the other hand to get the sound of a seashell. This stimulates the kidneys and the triple-warmer organs.

How to Use Deep Muscle Therapy for Arthritis

In Canada a woman has been curing arthritis patients for years with what she calls muscle therapy. Therese Pfrimmer discovered this technique by curing herself after becoming paralyzed from the waist down. She tells us that there is no such thing as a *dead* muscle or nerve. The muscles become tight from overwork. They become tense, the blood supply shuts off, and the muscles become sealed off from the rest of the circulation.

This theory is not unlike reflex massage except that you dig in deeper, reaching through to the very muscles that lie against the bone in many cases. Sometimes these muscles will feel like hard rocks that cannot be brought back to life. But all they need is to receive the circulation of blood back into them, and they will return to normal, and you will be free from the ravages of painful and crippling disease.

MUSCLES, NOT NERVES, CAUSE CRIPPLING

Muscles should be soft and supple, but in tests of the muscle tone of paralyzed people certain muscles are found to be tough, dry, and hardened; the muscle fibers are stuck together and can't be separated. Therese Pfrimmer says that the crippling problems are in the muscles and not the nerves. Paralysis sets in because the muscles become sealed off from the bloodstream. When fresh oxygenated arterial blood is sealed off, the muscles start to degenerate and become hardened. The muscles are also cut off from the flow of lymph—a fluid that lubricates the muscles and keeps them from sticking to each

30

other. Without lymph there is friction and different muscles that should be free and able to move separately stick together.

Deep muscle therapy can be used for seemingly incurable illnesses. It can be used along with reflex massage to bring faster and even more rewarding results, especially in cases where the muscles have become degenerated. I believe that no muscle or nerve is ever dead; it is just strangled by lack of circulation and *can* be brought back to life and health by releasing the flow of lymph and blood back into it. But exercise and physical therapy alone cannot cure a crippling condition where muscles have become hardened. They must be massaged, and the massage must be done in a certain way.

Suppose some of the muscles have been deprived of a supply of vital electrical energy for a long time. The blood supply has slowly been lessened to certain areas of the body. The muscles have become less and less pliable and more painful. When the muscles cannot move a joint, pain and inflammation occur because the muscles are pulling on the joint tissues. When you release the muscles, the joint will repair itself, and pain and stiffness will disappear. In cases such as this, it is often too late for reflexology alone to benefit, so we will turn to the sensational healing principle of deep muscle massage.

HOW DEEP MUSCLE MASSAGE HELPS ARTHRITIS

Here we will deviate a little from the way I have instructed you to use reflex massage. To help get the circulation back into degenerated muscles, we are going to have to reach in deep and massage them back to life. I believe that no muscle or nerve is *dead* as long as you are *alive*. But, after years of being denied the life-giving flow of blood and lymph, they may have become hard and fibrous. To get these muscles back into their natural state of pliability, we must massage them back to life. In some cases, it may not be easy and it may take time to get complete relief, but it will be worth your effort. In many cases, you will feel results almost immediately.

Now, to start using the muscle massage you will press with the fingers wherever the arthritis is bothering you. Take the fingers and press into or near the affected area of the arms or the legs or other parts of the body. Are the muscles soft and pliable, or are they hard against the bone? To massage these areas correctly, dig the fingers into the flesh and reach the muscle lying against the bone, if that is where it feels tight and hard. Start kneading across the muscles—not with them but across them, as if you were pulling across the strings of a guitar, only with a deep massaging motion. This may be painful, but it is the only way to get the flow of blood back into muscles that have become badly degenerated.

Therese Pfrimmer tells us that we must work on the second and third layers of muscles, not just the muscles lying under the skin which are usually treated by regular massage. Remember, we are not just pressing buttons here as in the technique of reflex massage.

THE IMPORTANCE OF THE ENDOCRINE SYSTEM

We look to the endocrine glands in treating the underlying cause of arthritis. When any one or more of these glands are not functioning to their full capacity, there is trouble elsewhere in the body. Look again at Diagram 2; then turn to Diagram 12 and notice where the endocrine reflexes are on the head. You will find the reflexes to the pituitary and the pineal glands located in the center of the forehead and under the nose. Gonad (sex gland) reflexes are at the top of the head and the center of the chin. The adrenal and pancreas reflexes are also located near the top of the head. Also see the reflex buttons to the triple warmer reflexes shown in Diagram 14.

Using all the fingers as shown in Photos 5, 7, 8, and 9, press these reflexes with a steady pressure, holding to a slow count of seven. Now, with the middle finger of each hand, press and massage each reflex button that feels sensitive to the touch. Try to follow the reflexes illustrated on the diagrams as much as possible.

Now, let us look at Diagrams 7 and 8 showing the location of the endocrine reflexes on the body. Press these with the fingers or a hand reflex massager, or stimulate a lot of these by using the helpful reflex roller.

HOW TO STIMULATE NATURAL CORTISONE

Cortisone is a drug used to stop pain. When we massage the reflexes to certain glands, we stimulate these glands into releasing a form of *natural* cortisone into the bloodstream. We are all aware of the damaging side effects that synthetic cortisone has on the body when it is injected. The natural cortisone produced by our glands alleviates pain quickly without any harmful side effects.

Review Diagram 6. Notice a point between the first and the second lumbar vertebrae near the lower part of the back. Press this point, using a gentle pressure to start, increasing it gradually for about seven seconds. This will cause a gland to secrete a natural human cortisone.

Most of you will not know exactly where the first and second lumbar vertebrae are located, but if you start by placing your fingers on the tailbone and then pressing gently on each vertebra, you will feel a very sensitive spot about three fingers' width up from the end of the spine. Use a press-and-hold on this, about three times, and your pain will vanish as if by magic. You may use this for any ailment in which cortisone is helpful. This is especially good for arthritis in various parts of the body, as well as asthma and bursitis.

Bursitis Alleviated

Dear Mrs. Carter,

Reflexology is the most wonderful and natural way of healing I ever dreamed of. I have been taking these treatments for about five years and have been giving them for over two years to friends and neighbors. What really made a believer out of me was this: I had bursitis in my shoulder and I had two pins in one ankle for over twenty years. The ankle was very sore. I had lots of pain and swelling. After two treatments my shoulder was fine, and after three treatments my ankle was much better. Now I have no trouble with bursitis at all.

—Mrs. N.P.

Another Arthritis Sufferer Helped

Dear Mrs. Carter,

I want to tell you of the wonderful results I have gotten from reflexology.

I had arthritis ever since I was seventeen years old and now I am forty-six years old; this is the first time that I am without pain. Plus, my husband was losing all his hair and after doing the hand reflexology as you directed, his hair stopped falling out and is now growing back. I want to thank you very much, and God bless you.

—I.A.

How to Use Reflexology to Relieve Back Pain

All practitioners recognize the importance that the spine has in the general health of the whole body. A great part of one's well-being depends on the condition of the spine. The largest percentage of back pain is caused from tension in the muscles that surround the spine. When undue strain is placed on a muscle somewhere in the back area, it tends to tighten and pull on certain vertebrae, causing the spine to be pulled out of alignment. We are all aware that the body can never function in perfect health if the spine is out of alignment.

LOW BACK PAIN IS THE LARGEST SINGLE MEDICAL COMPLAINT IN THE UNITED STATES

Many people in our country have suffered from this painful malady for years. They have gone to doctors and chiropractors without any lasting relief. When they finally searched out a reflexologist who understood the method of massaging the reflexes, in most cases they found permanent relief.

Back Pain Relieved All Over the World

I have received hundreds of letters from all over the world telling of the wonderful relief people have received from painful back problems. They used the simple but rewarding method of massaging the reflex-

34

es to the back that are located on their hands and on their feet. Now we will go a step further and show you how to use this wonderful healing method of massaging reflexes on other parts of the body, which will also bring almost instant relief from back pain.

Back Helped for Good

Dear Mrs. Carter,

I was troubled with painful back muscles for several weeks. Nothing seemed to help for long. One day, I decided I would try a different technique of reflex massage, since it had always helped me for other painful symptoms. I checked my hand with the chart and decided that I had not been massaging in the correct place. The muscles on the right side of my back were affected, so I felt for tender spots on the pad of my right hand below the little finger, and sure enough, I discovered some very tender places. After rubbing them a few minutes, the pain in my back lessened. In three days, all pain and tightness were gone and never returned. It pays to use your own testing along with the help of the charts when a problem doesn't clear up with ordinary directions. I truly believe that there is a reflex someplace that will alleviate pain and eliminate its cause, if we just search for it. I have proved this to be true. Thank you.

—Mrs. J.S.

Relief from Back Pain

Dear Mrs. Carter,

I am a twenty-one-year-old female who is employed in a job that requires me to stand and bend over all day. I have seen several chiropractors, but have not gotten much relief. Last Monday, I could barely walk, move, bend over, or turn my head because my lower back hurt so badly. My friend told me to try reflexology. I was willing to try anything so I went to see Mrs. K., and within fifteen minutes I felt like a new person. That afternoon I was able to shop and do housework, and most important of all I was able to go to work the next day, pain free! I was so happy with the results, I am now a firm believer in reflexology.

—C.N.

Reflexology Brings Instant Relief

Dear Mrs. Carter,

Three weeks ago, one of my students, a young woman in her late twenties, was suffering excruciating pain from an injured back. She dreaded taking the medication the doctor had given her for she suffered ill effects, and would not be able to attend school. I could not touch her in the school environment, so I told her to take off her shoes, and I directed her how to massage the response area to the spine. She had instant relief. She has been attending school every day since then, in perfect health. To me, the best investment I have made is the time I put into studying reflexology. It makes me happy to see the expression of relief and joy on the faces of those who have been restored to health.

—Ms. B.

How to Work the Tender Buttons

Let me explain how to work the reflexes in the hands and the feet to relieve many types of back pain.

You will note in Diagram 5 that the whole spinal column is located in the exact center of the body. Now look to the feet and note that from the big toe on the inside of the foot there is almost a replica of the spine. Follow this area with the fingers or a reflex device as it progresses along the foot to the heel. If you have any weakness in the spine, you will find very tender spots along this area. If the tenderness is near the toe, then the spine is weak between the shoulders. As it progresses toward the heel, you are following the spine down to the tailbone (coccyx). When you work on any of these tender places, you are stimulating a renewed life force into the part of the spine that for some reason is not getting a full supply of energy. When you work these tender buttons on your feet, it is like turning on an electric circuit that has been cut off from its source of power.

In the hands we find the same reflexes to the spine, but our blueprint of the electrical circuit of reflex buttons is moved to the forefinger and the bone that goes from the base of the finger to the wrist. See Photo 11. We also work on the bony structures of the thumb where it joins the wrist. This helps the lower back.

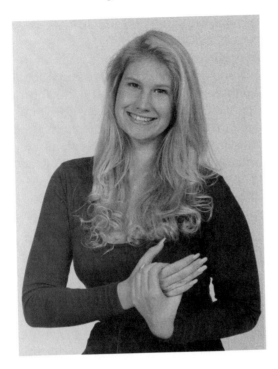

Photo 11: Position for massaging reflexes in the hands to overcome back problems.

Cure in a Few Minutes

Dear Mrs. Carter,

When my brother brought me to you, I was in so much pain from my back I could hardly walk. I had strained my lower back about a week before, and it kept getting worse instead of better. My family finally talked me into going to see you. In just a few minutes my pain was gone after you pressed a few reflexes in my back and then on the backs of my legs. Now any time I have a backache, I have my wife work on these reflexes like you showed us. We can't thank you enough.

—S.M.

WHY OTHER TREATMENTS SOMETIMES FAIL

When muscles are not loose and pliable, they can pull the bones out of place again (after a spinal adjustment) if they remain tight. In most cases, chiropractic adjustment helps, but if the back does not respond to adjustment, turn to reflex massage to relax and loosen up those tight muscles.

All muscles need fresh oxygenated blood and can't respond to nerve impulses without it. Tight muscles are starved for oxygen. So, let us first learn to loosen those muscles. When you massage the muscles to loosen them so that fresh oxygenated blood can flow into them, you are also reopening channels for the flow of life energy to the electrical system. The life force once more flows through all the circuits and brings nature's healing power into play. When you press on certain reflex buttons, you open channels through which the healing forces surge to malfunctioning areas of the body.

LOW BACK PAIN IS CAUSED BY TIGHT MUSCLES IN THE HAMSTRINGS

When the hamstring muscles in the backs of the legs become tight, they pull on the pelvis. You can see how this, in turn, pulls on all the muscles and tendons of the lower back. This places pressure on the spine and throws the back out of alignment, causing the discs to slip, rupture, or disintegrate.

Let us now learn how to massage these hamstring muscles to loosen them up and get the oxygenated blood flowing back through them. Sit on the edge of a chair, preferably a straight, hard chair. Relax one leg and place the fingers on the muscles of the thigh on the back of the leg. Press and pull the fingers across the muscles with one hand, then the other. Use the fingers of the other hand to pull across in the opposite direction. Do you feel any hard muscles? Dig in deeper and deeper as you search for a hard, bound muscle. Start at the buttocks and press and pull all the way to where the muscles end at the knee. When you find a hard, tight muscle, massage, press, and pull it. Remember, you are to pull the fingers *across* the muscle, not with it.

When you have finished with this leg, do the same massage on the other one. Remember, if you find any hard, tight muscles in this area, they must be worked out and become soft and pliable when relaxed. Your trouble may be caused by hard tight muscles lying very deep, even those next to the bone, so don't be afraid to massage deep. Work every tight area that you find. It could be quite painful in some cases at first.

If you have someone else to massage the hamstring muscles for you, then lie on a hard table or even the floor. After you get the muscles back to normal, you will find that the reflexes to the back will respond much more quickly, and you will get even better results than you had previously.

Feet Can Cause Back Problems

Some 20 percent of back pain is caused by flat feet. It can be corrected by wearing corrective shoes along with reflex massage. Experiment by wearing different shoes. Many times shoes are the cause of backaches.

Walking Is Beneficial to the Back

Walking is the best exercise for any back problems; it is nature's method of strengthening all the muscles in your body, especially your back muscles. It sends more blood and oxygen to every cell and tissue in your body, including the brain, eyes, and all internal organs. You may walk briskly, but there is no need to run. Jogging has proved to be harmful to 40 percent of those who jog.

A rebounder, which is a small trampoline, will prove to be very beneficial without harming the bone structure of the body and will give you many more benefits than jogging. Vitamin C has been proven to help many a backache.

Straighten Your Back with Foot Exercise

You can correct many ailments with the feet. When I was about seven years old some doctors came through the schools testing our health for various problems. They drew lines down my back and told me it was very crooked. They gave me exercises to do with my feet. In about a month they returned and drew lines on my back again. They were amazed to see how my back had straightened out.

Here are the exercises they gave me: Hold the feet straight out in front of the body, about ten inches apart. Curl the toes back toward the body as far as possible, then bring feet toward each other, so big toes touch. Now force down, holding your toes under as you take twenty steps, walking pigeon-toed. Relax and straighten feet out. Repeat one time then relax feet by shaking each one two or three times.

When you are barefoot, walk briskly around the room, taking four steps walking on toes and four steps walking on heels. Walk a total of twenty steps to strengthen the feet. Sometimes I walk on the outside of my feet, then on the inside. I still do these exercises to keep my back straight and strong.

Stair Climbing

Just a few words about this wonderful exercise. Stair climbing will burn calories and is an excellent workout for the whole body. It works the ankles so the lymphatic system is stimulated to boost the immune system. Your heart and lungs will benefit, comparable to a brisk run, swim, or bike ride. This may reduce stress by channeling it into a positive force. Smiling a very big smile while you exercise will stimulate your thymus.

How Reflexology Helps Back Pain Disappear

Dear Mrs. Carter,

I've learned that reflexology is simple, safe, and effective for anyone, anywhere, anytime. The dynamic healing force of reflexology can make you whole, can bring vigor, vitality, and beauty back into your life, and can help keep you free from illness and pain for the rest of your life if used properly. Reflex massage is therapeutic and can eliminate the cause and symptoms of sickness and pain from the whole body!

One Sunday morning while watching a baseball game on T.V. I felt a sharp pain in my lower back. I took my left foot and massaged the reflex button of the lower lumbar. In a few seconds my back pain suddenly disappeared. I massaged the right foot also. Now I know that reflexology really works.

Aloha and Mahalo!

—Mr. C.S., Hawaii

Relief from Back Pain and Sciatic Nerve

Dear Mrs. Carter,

First of all, I want to thank you for introducing me to reflexology. I read all your books. It has helped me cure my back pain and sciatic condition. I feel great and stay that way by using reflexology.

One day while at work one of my co-workers was not feeling very well. He told me his back went out again and he was getting pains down his leg. He told me he was going to see a chiropractor after work. I gently applied pressure to the reflex just below the hip (where the back pocket of his trousers is located). He was immediately relieved.

At lunch time, I gave him another quick reflex treatment. He felt so good that he told me he wasn't going to see the chiropractor after work!

—Mr. D.T.

How to Banish Bronchitis

VITAMIN C, THE MIRACLE VITAMIN

Vitamin C is one of the miracle vitamins in use today. It is inexpensive and available in health food stores, drugstores, and even in grocery stores. Vitamin C is lauded for its wonderful healing power for nearly every illness, including heart disease, strokes, and arthritis.

When vitamin C was first brought to my attention, it was described as preventing and curing colds. I immediately started to use it to stop colds before they actually got started.

Vitamin C Cures Chronic Bronchitis

One day Mrs. G., a friend I was visiting, told me of her family's cold problems. Every winter they spent several weeks in the hospital with flu and congested lungs. Gene, about nine years old, had suffered with bronchitis all his life. I told her about vitamin C and its healing properties, especially for colds. She said she would try it. A few months later, I again went to visit Mrs. G. and she told me what happened with the vitamin C that she had bought. She said that she placed the bottle on the table, but no one took any of the tablets.

One day, Mrs. G. noticed that the vitamin bottle on the table was empty, so she asked Gene about this. He said that since she had told him, "They are good for you and will make you well," he figured he would take them all and get well all at once—and he did get well all at once!

The following winter was one of the worst for colds and flu. Mrs. G. told me that they had all spent weeks in the hospital with colds and bronchial infections—but not Gene. He never had a cold or even a sniffle all winter long.

The next time I saw Gene he was in his twenties, and was a big, healthy, strong man who had never had a recurrence of bronchitis since the time he took the whole bottle of vitamin C.

I would not advise anyone to take an overdose of any vitamin, but in clinical studies they are proving that megadoses of vitamins are the answer to many puzzling health problems that modern medication will not cure.

Vitamins A and C reduce the damage smoking causes the body. If you can't quit smoking, take more vitamins A and C.

The late Paavo Airola, a noted nutritionist, said that vitamin C is involved in virtually all the functions of your body. It helps your body to protect itself against every stress and every condition threatening your health.

Dr. M. Higuchi, a Japanese researcher, tells us that his studies show a definite relationship between vitamin C levels in the diet and hormone production of the sex glands. He says that older people, particularly, need larger amounts of vitamin C to assure adequate sex hormone production.

When taking any vitamin or mineral tablets, I powder the tablets for better assimilation. To do this, lay the tablet between two sheets of waxed paper and crush with a hammer until it is powdered. Sprinkle on food or put into a milk or a drink. I suggest that you experiment on your own to find out how you like to take it best. Some vitamins are available in powdered and liquid form, others are made with natural flavors and are chewable.

GARLIC, A MIRACLE FOOD

I must not leave out the importance of garlic. It is known as a miracle vegetable. It has been used for thousands of years by various races and civilizations. Early Egyptians and Hebrews considered garlic a food endowed with divine properties—and it really is. Garlic is rich in several food chemicals as well as vitamins A, B, C, and D. (Vitamin D is the sunshine vitamin so necessary for existence.) It is also rich in sulfur and iodine. All these help to stimulate the liver and kidneys, eliminate worms from children and pets, and relieve rheumatic and arthritic conditions and many other ailments.

Reflexology for Bronchitis

Dear Mrs. Carter,

I know that everything you say in your books is true. I use so many of your methods to help friends and loved ones and myself. I will tell you of one experience I had.

One morning, I got up with a very bad cough. I was gagging and was very sick, so I went to a doctor. After looking at my throat and X-raying my chest, he said I had bronchitis. I informed my father-in-law of my problem and he used reflexology treatments on me as described in your book. I went back to the doctor in a few days and he said that I was well. Now, when I get sick, I go to my father-in-law and he makes me well. Everyone, young and old, should have your reflexology books in their home library.

Thank you.

—Mrs. M.N.

Treating Coughs and Colds with Reflexology

Colds and flu usually start with a sore throat, so let's cure the sore throat before it turns into something worse.

If I feel the slightest warning of sore throat, the first thing that I do is the lion posture from yoga. This simple posture stops a sore throat before it gets started. See Photo 12. Get down on your knees, sit back on your heels, place the hands on the knees, and spread the fingers as far apart as you can. Inhale a deep breath, and as you exhale the breath, stick out your tongue, straining to reach the chin with the tip of the tongue until you almost gag. Stiffen your fingers and bug your eyes out as you become very tense. Hold this position of tension for a few seconds, then relax. Repeat this posture four or five times, and you will be amazed to feel almost immediate relief from the sore throat. The lion posture rushes an extra supply of blood to the affected area. It tones and strengthens the muscles and ligaments in the throat.

A Yoga Posture Helps a Child

It is truly amazing how quickly this method stops a sore throat for all ages. I had my three-year-old granddaughter do this posture one day when she complained of her throat hurting. We made a game out of the posture and all got on the floor and did it with her. When she got up, she said, "I don't have an ow-ey in my neck anymore, Mommy." That was the end of the sore throat. My daughter was amazed even though she had been taught to use this posture since she was a young

45

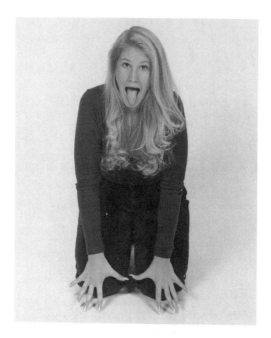

Photo 12: Kneeling position to cure a sore throat.

child. She said, "We get so involved with doctors and advertised drugs, we forget the true and simple healing methods of nature."

Healing in Strange Places

I have taught this posture to many of my friends, some in very odd places—like in the rest room of a large resort. A young woman with a bad sore throat was going to cut her vacation short and go home. She told me, "We planned this vacation for months, went to a lot of work finding the right person to stay with the children, got reservations almost a year ahead, and now, this! We really needed to get away by ourselves for a while. We have a whole two weeks and have only been here two days." I asked her if she would try an odd exercise to help cure the sore throat in a hurry.

I had her put her sweater on the floor to kneel on and showed her how to do the lion posture. She did it several times, and when she got up, she looked at me in amazement. She felt her throat, swallowed a few times, and said it felt completely well. I showed her the reflexes on the feet and the hands, told her to massage any spots that showed tenderness, and advised her to do the lion posture whenever she felt

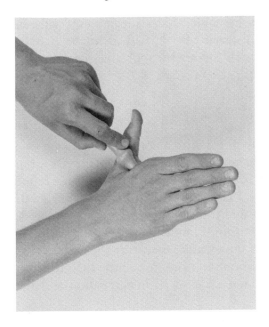

Photo 13: Using reflex hand probe to stimulate many parts of the body— great for pain relief, insomnia, and anxiety.

she needed it. I also told her to get some apple cider vinegar if she could. If this was not possible, any kind of vinegar would do. She should dilute it with water and gargle often, swallowing a little each time she gargled.

I don't know when I have ever seen anyone so elated. She hugged me and cried with joy. She said that she would call home and tell her baby-sitter what to do with the children if they developed sore throats. We saw her and her husband several times after that, and they were acting like happy newlyweds.

USING HAND REFLEXES

The reflex for the throat is located on the lower part of the thumb where it fastens onto the hand and all of that area including the web between the fingers. See Photo 13. This also holds true with the reflexes to the throat on the feet. Search for any tender spots anywhere on the big toe where it joins the foot. I have stopped many a sore throat by massaging this particular area. I find this so, especially, on very small children who cannot do the postures and people who are not able to kneel on the floor for the lion posture. See Photo 12.

There is healing benefit in apple cider vinegar, especially in destroying germs. In Dr. D. C. Jarvis's book, *Folk Medicine*, he tells of the uses for and cures brought about by applying cider vinegar. One of them is its ability to cure strep throat.

An Unusual Remedy

I brought my eight-year-old granddaughter home to our ranch one summer. Her mother said the girl had been to a doctor for strep throat, but that she had been cured by medication. We were home about two days when I noticed that she was having a hard time swallowing. I looked in her throat and found it covered with white nodules. I knew the strep was back again. I immediately started giving her a mixture of two teaspoons of apple cider vinegar in a glass of water. I had her gargle this every half-hour and swallow a little each time. In a very short time, the throat was clear of all inflammation and the strep germs never returned.

EXPLORING THE TONGUE

Using a tongue probe is also very helpful in curing a sore throat. Just press the back of the tongue with a reflex tongue massager, feeling for tender buttons on the tongue. Some of these can be very sore, but remember what we say in reflexology: "If it hurts, rub it out." Since this is a sensitive reflex area for many malfunctions of the body, be sure to keep a check on any tender spots that might appear on the tongue. See Photo 14.

HELP FOR OTHER SYMPTOMS

Now that we have learned to eliminate one of the first signs of a cold, let us go to the other symptoms, such as sneezing and coughs.

When one has developed a bad cold, it is wise not to give complete reflexology treatments. A cold usually indicates that impurities have accumulated in the system and that the body is trying to clean house by expelling these harmful toxic substances. When we massage certain reflexes, we are helping the body throw off poisons and taxing certain glands and organs, causing them to do extra work in helping

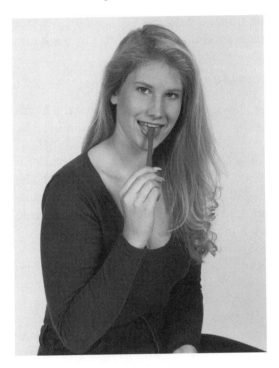

Photo 14: Shows reflex tongue probe ready to be used on the reflexes on the back of the tongue.

the body clean house. So, the only reflexes we will work on during a cold are the pituitary reflex, which is located in the center of the big toe and the thumb, and the throat reflexes. Also, we can press and massage the reflexes to the lungs to help them utilize an added supply of oxygen.

You will see the special reflex buttons for the lungs as you study Diagrams 7 and 8. Press this whole area if you find tender spots on or near the reflex points. Also, search for tender reflexes in the ears and the body warmer buttons on the head. See Diagrams 14 and 15.

If you want to abort a cold before it gets started, take a coffee enema. I have done this many times, and it really works. Use about three teaspoons of instant coffee to a quart of warm water or make a pot of regular coffee and use it. It is said that it stimulates the liver. Do not use a coffee enema at night; it may keep you awake. Use honey instead.

Vinegar and honey are good remedies to take orally, and don't forget the power of the onion and the magic healing properties of garlic. We all know that we must take a large amount of vitamin C to stop a cold or to help get over one quickly. Take a lot of lemons, but not oranges or grapefruit. Massage the pituitary reflexes to lower a fever.

How a Bad Cough Was Stopped Instantly

While I was in a large hotel in Hawaii, I noticed that one of the maids had a very bad cough. She hardly stopped coughing between breaths. When we went out into the hall, I walked up to her and said, "Here, hold your finger like this." I showed her how to squeeze the joint near the end of her middle finger with the fingers of the opposite hand. She looked very puzzled and doubtful until an older Hawaiian maid came and said, "You do what she says, she knows." So the girl did as I told her and she stopped coughing almost immediately.

When we came back several hours later, she greeted me with the greatest enthusiasm—she couldn't thank me enough. There was no sign of the cough that had been troubling her earlier. We were there for several days, and I never heard her cough again.

I hope that you will pass the sensational principle of simple reflex massage on to anyone who might meet with a hard-to-overcome health problem. And then tell them to pass the information on to others. In this way, you will light one more candle to send out healing beams to a sick and suffering world.

How Reflexology Cures Headaches

Headaches occur for many reasons, some due to a specific health problem such as flu, digestive problems, depression, eyestrain, sinus trouble, hay fever and other allergies, and stress. When using reflexology, you will work on the reflex point that corresponds to the part of the body causing the pain. Millions of people turn to drugs to get temporary relief. Now, you can turn to nature and reflexology and learn sure, quick ways to stop a headache almost immediately. You can do it yourself any place the headache strikes—at home, in the office, at a party, while camping, and so on. Because reflexology tends to heal the whole body by opening up closed electrical lines, it prevents the headache from recurring.

Look at Diagrams 12, 13, and 14. No wonder the head can ache in so many places. Notice all the reflex buttons on the head and face. When you think that each one of these is connected to an electrical channel that leads to some part of your body, you can readily understand why the head can ache.

USING HAND REFLEXES

Let us start with the reflexes in the hands. These are the simplest, easiest reflexes to reach in any emergency. Since the reflexes in the thumbs represent the head area, first massage the thumb reflexes. With the thumb of the opposite hand, start pressing on the center of the pad of the thumb; then squeeze the sides of the thumb by pressing each side of the nail. With a firm pressure, massage just below the

51

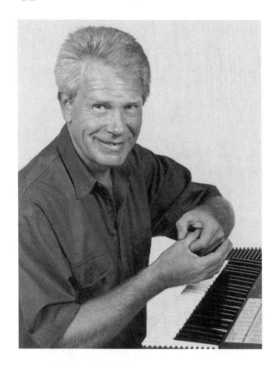

Photo 15: Organist massages reflexes in the thumb to relax nerves and stop a headache.

thumbnail on top of the thumb, searching for tender buttons. Cover the complete thumb with searching massage; remember, do not rub the skin, but the reflexes *under* the skin. If you don't find a sore spot on one thumb, change hands and give the other thumb the same massage. When you do find an "ouch" spot, massage it for several minutes or until the head stops aching. This works nine times out of ten. See Photo 15.

If the headache persists, place the thumb on the web of the opposite hand between the thumb and forefinger. Pinch and massage this whole area, clear up to where you feel the bones come together, searching for tender buttons. See Diagrams 12A and 12D and Photo 13. This reflex stimulates many parts of the body, so if you find an "ouch" spot here, be sure to rub it out. If you can't find a sore spot here, change hands and do the same to the opposite hand. Since this is one of the crucial reflex buttons for the whole body, it is a good idea to keep this area free from sore spots at all times.

If the headache *still* persists, press and massage the reflexes in the center of both hands, searching for tender buttons. The magic massager will be useful here—it should be used every day to help keep these reflexes stimulated and the electrical life lines open to every part of the body.

Using Foot Reflexes

You will find that massaging the reflexes of the feet works miracles, not only for headache but for any other health problem that you might have. Massage all the reflexes in each foot, searching for tender reflex buttons. You may find the reflexes in the feet to be more sensitive than anywhere else on the body. I believe these reflexes in the feet to be most powerful of all in their ability to stimulate the healing life force to every part of your body by opening up closed or clogged electrical lines.

This is why I so highly recommend a reflex foot massager. It is easy to use while you are watching television, talking on the phone, or sitting anywhere. See Photos 16 and 17. It will really stimulate the *healing universal life force* within every part of your body and touch the malfunctioning area that is causing the painful headache. If you haven't already overcome the headache, let us go on to other reflex buttons.

Photo 16: Position for using a reflex foot massager to energize the healing life force into most parts of the body.

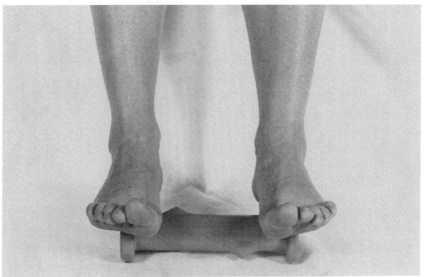

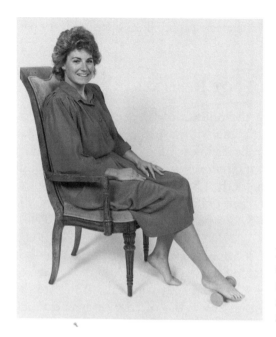

Photo 17: Shows comfortable position while using a reflex foot massager to help nature rejuvenate the body naturally.

I received a letter from one of my students who was successful in relieving her friend from terrible headache pain. Here is the letter:

Dear Mrs. Carter,

One of my close friends had been to a neurologist and many other doctors, and had many tests to find out how she could cure a very bad headache. Unfortunately, she did not have any success until I was able to persuade her to allow me to work on the inside of her second toe where it joins the foot next to the big toe. After only a few times of working this reflex point, her headache stopped. She is now spreading around the wonderful news of her healing.

God bless and many thanks,

—N.G.

DEALING WITH FREQUENT HEADACHES

Massaging the Head

Look at Diagram 13; see the button called the medulla oblongata at the base of the skull. This button is important in addressing sev-

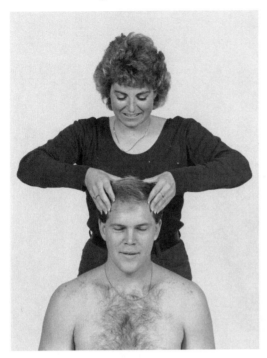

Photo 18: Position for massage of the reflexes in the head by another person.

eral health complaints that are mainly caused by stress. This is what we call a stress button. Pressing it will bring relief to several health complaints besides a headache. Since its location makes it hard to find and control the pressure needed, it will be more convenient if you use the hand reflex massager. You do not need to press very hard on this particular reflex, just firmly enough to feel the pressure in your head.

Look at Photos 5, 7, 8, 9, and 18 to see how the fingers are being pressed on many areas of the head at once. Use a light but firm pressure as you move the fingers onto different reflexes with a slightly rotating massage. Remember, you are massaging reflexes under the skin, not the skin itself. If you find any reflexes painful to the touch, massage them for a few minutes. Massage the reflexes around the ears, searching for tender reflexes. There is a reflex on the ear that has been known to relieve certain types of headaches. First, you will need to look at Diagram 15, noticing the reflexes to the neck, forehead, and back of head. These basic reflex points are on the cartilage along the back side and bottom of the ear opening. Hold the thumb behind the

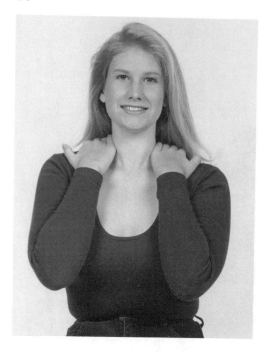

Photo 19: Position for massaging reflexes in the neck and shoulders.

ear and press your index or middle finger into these points (one finger will reach all points as you move it in a pressing, soothing circular motion). Then press and work the ear lobe, gently if the headache is mild and vigorously if the pain is intense. Keep massaging on down the side of the neck to the shoulders and along the top of the shoulders. See Photo 19. Massage all the muscles in the back of the neck to relieve tension that may be slowing the circulation to the brain, eyes, and other organs within the head. See Photo 6.

Using the Heel of Your Hands for Additional Pressure

If your fingers do not have enough strength to work the reflex points on your head, you may want to use the heel of your hands. Be careful when using this exercise, not to press too hard, as one usually has more strength than they realize when using this type of pressure. You can use the heel of one hand at a time, or you can clasp hands together (see Photo 20) behind your head—using the heels of your hands to work and press the reflex points. You will be able to reach many reflex points with this technique.

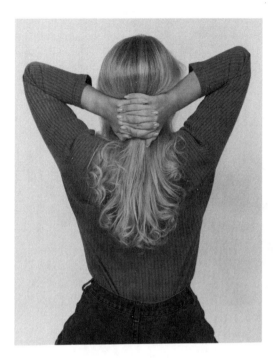

Photo 20: For additional pressure use the heel of hands to stimulate reflexes in back of head.

Bend Head Forward for Quick Relief

Now I will tell you another quick way to release pressure from the head area. Bend your head forward, working the reflexes on your head. Press lightly over the whole head with your fingers or knuckles, in a slow shampooing motion. Start at the top and work down. If you find tender reflexes, work these points for 15 to 30 seconds, then move on. Go back and forth, covering the entire head—each time you may add additional pressure, but never too hard or you may cause bruising.

Move your hands away from your body and give them a slight shake; this will drain tension away from the head. Repeat twice.

Relieving Headaches Caused by Eyestrain

If eyestrain is causing a headache you will work the reflex buttons for the eyes, which you will find on each foot at the base of the second and third toes or on the hands at the base of the index and middle finger of each hand. See Diagrams 3 and 5.

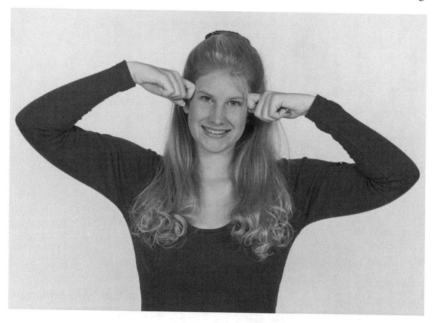

Photo 21: Use knuckles to relieve tension headaches. Knuckles work well for those who have weak fingers or long fingernails.

Another reflex button can be found just above, and on both sides of, the bridge of the nose. Slightly above the eyes, just below the underside of the eyebrow, use middle fingers and simultaneously work buttons.

The most common reflex point on the head is found at the outer side of the eyes, at the temples. Reach up and rub these points simultaneously with your middle fingers. If you have long fingernails, or your fingers are weak, you can use your knuckles. See Photo 21.

OTHER METHODS FOR RELIEVING HEADACHES

You may need to change your diet by eating lots of fresh vegetables and fruits, avoiding sugar and chocolate and (for some people) coffee and dairy products. *Don't overeat.* This is the most common sin against health committed by the American people. We eat too much. I can remember people saying that my grandparents didn't eat enough to keep a bird alive. They lived healthy lives to the ages of 99 and 103.

The late Edgar Cayce told many of his people to sit with the back straight and bring the chin forward to touch the chest, then tilt the head back as far as possible to help open the flow of blood in the pipelines leading to and from the head. I knew a woman who did this one hundred times every day, and she threw away her glasses. Don't do this more than five times at first, or you will develop a headache from tight and sore muscles.

One of the best ways to relieve a headache is to do a lot of walking, especially if you do it in the fresh air. Be sure to wear good shoes. The theory seems to be when we exercise, the lungs process more oxygen, which will increase circulation and ease tension. Aerobics, walking, deep breathing, and reflexology all are good avenues to avoiding tension headaches.

Another person wrote to tell me that the best treatment for them, along with the use of reflexology, is a good fifteen-minute hand or foot soak. She claimed that this always seemed to work for her. This does work for some people, as the hands or feet become hot, the body temperature raises in this area of the body...which ultimately brings the blood flowing down to this part of the body and away from the head to release built-up tension.

I have given you many ways to banish your headaches forever. You will not need to do all these techniques; choose the ones that seem to help you the most, and live the rest of your life free from pain.

How to Cure a Migraine Headache

If you feel that you have what is called a migraine headache, the first thing to do is look for the cause. Many people have suffered for years from terrible headaches, only to discover they were caused by an allergy to a simple household item or by an additive in food. Eliminate this cause by experimenting. Some migraines are caused by the spine or the neck being out of adjustment. Many headaches are caused by air pollution.

My daughter had terrible headaches for years; the muscles on the back of her neck would tighten up, stopping the circulation of blood to her head. She moved out of the valley into the mountains and her headaches stopped almost completely. When she went to town in the valley, she always came home with a terrible headache. Reflex massage helped, but we couldn't get at the cause until we discovered that the

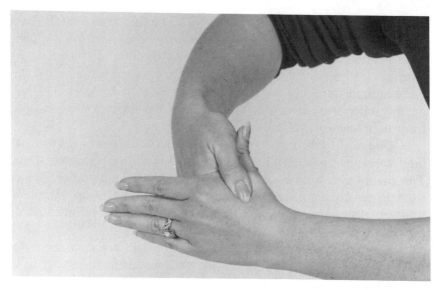

Photo 22: Pressure point to relieve pain in many parts of the body, including abdominal pain, headaches and cramps.

culprit was the smog. It had been causing what we thought were migraine headaches.

I know of many people who have rid themselves of what they called migraine headaches by using reflex massage. After you have pressed the reflex buttons on your body, including the reflexes on the hands and feet, search the neck and head for tender buttons that will give you a clue to the cause of your pain. Work on all the reflexes involved. Massage all tenderness out. Keep the thymus active by tapping it often, and smile a lot. See Photo 1.

Especially massage the medulla oblongata at the back of the head. See Diagram 13. Also massage the reflex buttons halfway between the medulla and the ears. See Photo 6. Massage the pain reflexes, the web between the thumb and forefinger (see Photos 13 and 22) and also between the large toe and the second toe. See Diagrams 6A, 6D, and 6E. Massage the reflexes to the stomach on the hands, feet, and body. See Diagrams 3, 5, 7, and 8.

The herb "feverfew" is very effective in stopping migraine headaches for many people. The recommended amount is one tablet, three times a day.